Expecting Grace

The Miraculous Survival Story of a Hyperemesis Gravidarum Pregnancy

Leah A. Highfill

Expecting Grace

The Miraculous Survival Story of a Hyperemesis Gravidarum Pregnancy

by Leah A. Highfill

embracingrace.com

Cover design and interior layout by Jeff & Joy Miller at Five J's Design. http://fivejsdesign.com

Dedication

For Jonathan, the most dedicated and loving of husbands. Thank you for walking with me through some of the darkest days of our married life. Thank you for being a wonderful father to our miracle child. Thank you for encouraging me to follow new dreams that Hyperemesis can't take away.

Table of Contents

Introduction

"It's a boy!" I remember being shocked. My husband, Jonathan, and I had both strongly believed our first instincts that the baby would be a girl.

More than that, though, I just couldn't believe that our baby was alive.

One...two...nine...ten. All the fingers and toes were there. He was healthy- simply amazing. A million thoughts flooded my mind as the past nine months flashed through my consciousness. It was hard to believe that it had been "only" nine months; it really had seemed like nine years.

To this day, that nine-month period seems like the longest section of my life by far. It seems even longer than my childhood in some ways. Maybe it's because the memories are so vivid, leaving just about every waking minute of that time period fresh in my mind, as if it happened yesterday. Not only physical adjustments remain; that season in our lives was emotionally traumatic. Girlhood dreams of childbearing were shattered. Having a family was no longer a matter of excited planning—it was a matter of life and death.

It was a time of making very difficult decisions and of trusting God with the outcome.

Since that time, I've come to realize that I'm not alone. Although a very small group of women suffer with the same condition, awareness is very minimal.

I survived, by God's grace and many miracles, a life threatening pregnancy. Furthermore, I recognize that there are many women in our world who have suffered difficult pregnancies because of various complications. I desire for this book to be a source of encouragement for these very women. Pregnancy is a very emotionally precious time. When things go wrong, we are tempted to worry, and often our "having a baby" dreams get muddled. Sometimes, as in my experience, those dreams have to die. God has other dreams. And along the path of grief, there is grace. I didn't always know it or feel it. Most days were a fog of "what on earth is happening to me?" thoughts. But looking back, I know that each moment was tenderly guarded and guided by my loving heavenly Father. He was weaving a new dream. And although it took me several years to offer my "thank you" to God, He has indeed brought me to that place of humbleness and blessing—that place of non-reversible comfort.

And this is what brings me to this page, seven years later, to tell my story of a pregnancy miracle.

What is Hyperemesis Gravidarum?

Hyperemesis Gravidarum—do you know what it is? Based on statistics, it is probably an unfamiliar medical term to you. But perhaps you know someone who had it, or you had it yourself, but you didn't know it had a name. The fact that you have your hands on this book may mean that you are part of the statistical 1-2% of women who suffer with HG during pregnancy.

You wish you didn't know what it was. Furthermore, you wish people understood that you aren't just "morning sick," that crackers don't help, that you do want the baby, that you are not crazy, but that you have a serious pregnancy disease. You wish they understood how desperately you need support.

So what is Hyperemesis Gravidarum? In my own words (and from my experience), it is a life-threatening pregnancy disease characterized by unrelenting nausea, vomiting, and extreme dehydration that often lasts the entire length of the pregnancy. Unlike morning sickness which eases off as the pregnancy progresses, HG gets worse as the hormone levels increase. It is, by a simpler definition, a type of rare intolerance of abnormally high levels of the pregnancy hormone. About 1 in 300 women suffer with this misunderstood disease.

The only known cure? Giving birth.

The first purpose of this book is to be a testimony to God's grace as I tell the true story of our struggle and survival of our first pregnancy. It is a story of difficult events, but shining through the trauma are the miracles and the blessings that make this story worth telling. We watched God do wonders on our behalf—wonders that often left us and even our doctors in awe. We know that we have not been the only ones to experience HG, and we hope our story will inspire and encourage others who have gone through the same experience, who are going through it now, and who will face it in the future.

The second purpose of this book is to raise awareness of HG. More people need to know what HG is! It is not just the women who suffer (often in silence) who need more awareness and support. Husbands suffer. Other children suffer. Extended families and friends need to be aware of the effects of HG, so that they can better support someone they know who is going through it.

Most of the time when my pregnancies come up in a conversation, it goes like this:

"How many children do you have?" asks New Aquaintance.

"Two—a boy and a girl" says me.

"Do you plan to have any more?" asks New Aquaintance.

"No, I had HG while I was pregnant, and it would be life-threatening to have any more," says me.

"You had what?" asks New Aquaintance, and then I know I have a lot of explaining to do.

Wouldn't it be nice if the conversation went like this (and on rare occasions, it has!):

"How many children do you have?"

"Two—a boy and a girl,"

"Do you plan to have any more?"

"No, I had HG while I was pregnant..."

"Oh wow! I'm so sorry!" or "Oh! You had that too?!" or "I have a friend who had that. It was horrible."

When the conversation goes like that, an instant connection is made between two women who understand each other. When we meet someone who doesn't understand, it is almost like we can't explain it the right way. "I was really sick" just doesn't cut it. It has to be someone who has experienced it to truly understand. I'm wondering maybe, just maybe, if more of us told our stories, would more people understand? Would more people try to find a cure?

It's time to end the silence of HG; it's time to tell our stories, to raise awareness, and to inspire each other with the strength of survival!

1 - A Normal Beginning

On May 14, 2005, I married my best friend. We, like most couples on their wedding day, didn't have much thought for the negative parts of our vows: "...for worse...in sickness...for poorer." Naturally, on that happy day, we were looking forward to a bright future. The knowledge that trouble will come is present in the mind, but somehow on that day it is nearly impossible to think of what those troubles might be.

And so it was for us. Our wedding went perfectly, and soon we found ourselves heading to Canada for our honeymoon. While there, we candidated at a church that was considering hiring my husband to be their youth pastor. By the time our honeymoon was over, we both knew for sure that this was where God wanted us to minister.

After returning home, we spent an enjoyable summer in North Carolina. As fall approached, we began packing our belongings in preparation for our big move to Canada. God answered many prayers as we prepared. We met deadlines for obtaining our passports and received on time a much-needed letter for border crossing. We prayed and watched God provide a large amount of money needed to rent the moving truck. Little did we know that some of these "small" miracles would be the things we would cling to later to remind ourselves that God is faithful!

On October 17, we packed the truck, said goodbye to our friends and family, and made the week-long trip to Canada, the new place we would call home.

I have one vivid memory of the day we moved into the parsonage. After setting down some boxes in a bedroom, one of the men who was helping us move asked, "Will you be needing that?" while pointing to a crib that was already in the house. I replied with a smile and without any thought, "Nope, we won't be needing that!"

2 – Faith or Fear?

"Beloved, think it not strange concerning the fiery trial which is to try you, as though some strange thing happened unto you: but rejoice, inasmuch as ye are partakers of Christ's sufferings; that, when his glory shall be revealed, ye may be glad also with exceeding joy." 1 Peter 4:12-13

One day in early November, we were having a devotional time together from a book we had been given as a wedding gift. It was a small, hardcover book entitled "Daily Light." It consisted of daily, topical readings for each morning and evening. On this particular day, the topic was trials. For some reason, these two verses from 1 Peter just jumped out at me. But instead of blessing me, the verses nagged at me, as if they were a shadow of things to come in our lives. I remember turning off the vacuum one day and telling Jonathan that I felt afraid, and that I had this weird feeling that something majorly negative was about to happen in our lives. I tried to push it out of my mind, but it continued to bother me.

A few weeks later, when I landed in the hospital for the first time, my mind raced back to those verses. God had begun testing our faith as a couple. Looking back, I realize now that my trust in God was not very strong. Often I find that when a verse of Scripture strikes fear into my heart, it is because I don't trust my heavenly Father in that area of my life. Today when I read those verses, I don't feel fear, but joy! Through the trial of a life-threatening pregnancy, and through other trials after that, we have been privileged to see God molding us to be more like Him. It seems unthinkable to compare our sufferings with those of Christ, yet He wants us to experience a certain close fellowship that only comes through earthly sufferings, as we allow Him to change us. While this story is primarily a medical one, it is also a spiritual story of the personal work of God in our lives.

3 - *The Day That Changed All Days*

Wednesday, November 23, 2005, was the day that changed all days for us. On my home pregnancy test, the positive sign showed up bright and clear. Our move to Canada had preoccupied most of our time and thoughts for the past two months, so we were somewhat surprised to learn that a certain small someone would be entering our lives. I should have known, though, as a few months earlier I had to go off of birth control because it made me violently ill. Now it makes sense to me, since birth control basically mimics the pregnancy hormone. My body just could not tolerate it.

On Saturday, November 26, I had the first inkling of not feeling well. We were at a

Christmas social at church, and I was standing up during a game. All of a sudden I felt very weak in my muscles. I remember thinking, "I need to sit down or I'm going to faint." I stayed pretty low-key the rest of the evening. "This is normal," I told myself, never imagining the nightmare that lay ahead.

Early the next morning, Sunday, I woke up very sick. We were hosting missionaries for the weekend, and they ended up hosting themselves! I never saw them again until five years later, and we actually had a good laugh about what happened that weekend. I missed church, and everyone found out by default that I was pregnant. Using hindsight, I now know that when you have HG, you have to announce the pregnancy right away, or you will never have a chance to. The only other option is to announce by being admitted to the hospital—now isn't that creative?!

By early Monday morning, it was obvious that my morning sickness no longer deserved the title of normal. I was very sick and weak, and even a drop of ginger ale only stayed down for a few seconds. It literally bounced. I was also experiencing sharp pains on my right side. So just to be safe, we went to the hospital, which was an hour away. Being in the car was torture; the constant movement only aggravated the already intense nausea, and I was so weak I could barely sit up.

Our first introduction to the socialized healthcare system was a real eye-opener. I was expecting immediate care, especially since I was (a) pregnant and (b) severely dehydrated from almost non-stop sickness for the past 24 hours. I thought 24 hours was a long time to be sick. I had a lot to learn. The nurse put me in a curtained off section of the outpatient department, and informed me that there was nothing they could do for me until the doctor had seen me.

"Ok," I thought, "That won't be too long."

But hours passed and I didn't even receive an IV, much less any medication to ease the nausea. Finally, about 12 hours later, a doctor appeared. He was foreign and very hard to understand when he talked. Furthermore, he got quite agitated if people couldn't get what he was saying immediately. However, he ordered an IV, some Gravol, blood work, and an ultrasound. After 36+ hours without fluid, that IV felt so good. I could literally feel that cool liquid rushing into my veins. The Gravol too brought instant relief from nausea; but it left me with a bad headache. At that point, though, a headache was a welcome exchange for the other symptoms!

An ultrasound was performed that evening almost immediately upon the doctor's orders. Water never tasted so good, although it was difficult to get enough down (and keep it there) to make the nurses happy. I watched the screen carefully as the ultrasound technician guided her instrument across my flat stomach. She didn't say anything (not even small talk, which would have eased my nerves considerably!), but proceeded to do an internal ultrasound to try to see more. I thought it was odd that I still couldn't see anything.

"But then," I thought, "I'm not trained to read ultrasounds."

The nurse turned the screen away and I knew there was something she didn't want me to see. I was returned to my curtained section in the outpatient ward.

4 – The Mystery

Around 6:00 PM, the doctor came in with his reports.

"There is no baby," he said, "just an empty sack."

I was confused—stunned even, not by this news, but by everything that had happened in the last 40 hours, now to be complicated by an ultrasound report like this. The doctor went on to say that he feared I was having an ectopic pregnancy, especially given how much pain I was in, and the fact that my HCG hormone levels were so high. Based on my dates, they had determined that I was about five weeks into the pregnancy. Since an ectopic pregnancy can be life-threatening to the mother, the doctor decided to admit me for a week of observation in case something should happen. The thought of a hospital stay terrified me, but common sense won over. Our home was an hour from the hospital, so we knew it was the most practical and safe thing to do.

An orderly named Jacob appeared to take me upstairs to my new room on the maternity floor. Jacob was such a kind man, and proved to be a source of comfort to us in the months that followed. He always seemed to appear just when we needed something. He had a ready smile and a helpful attitude. We arrived at my room, where he locked my bed in place and patted my hand. Behind the curtain of my semi-private room, my roommate was tending her newborn baby. I tried to fast-forward my mind to my own day like that, but my brain refused. One of the weirdest feelings I've ever had ensued as I settled into my bed.

"Am I pregnant or not?" I thought, "How can one be *in between* or *sort of* pregnant?"

My husband and I prayed together, committing our situation to God, and asking Him for some clear answers soon.

The next day, Tuesday, more blood work was done. The results showed that my HCG hormone levels had skyrocketed even higher during the night. So my doctor ordered another ultrasound for that afternoon. Much to everyone's surprise, there was a tiny heart beating away! We couldn't believe it. To this day, this part of our story remains a mystery to us. Why couldn't they find one just hours earlier? It was as if God had just placed a baby in there overnight while I slept.

5 – The Miscarriage

By Tuesday evening, I was having pain again on my right side. The doctor on call came in and examined me, pushing and prodding all over so he could figure out the cause of my discomfort. He didn't know what it could be, so once again we were left to our own confused selves. About an hour after he left the room, I started spotting, then bleeding more heavily. I knew what was happening and rang for the nurse. She kindly sympathized with me while I cried. (Looking back, I am surprised at how open the nurses were about it being a miscarriage, given the fact that no tests had been done to confirm it.) They made sure that I wasn't blaming myself that the baby didn't survive.

My feelings at this point were hard to be understood, even by my own heart. Having been in limbo about whether or not there really was a baby in there, I had only had a few hours to adjust to the news that there was one indeed. Now it seemed, again, that there wasn't one. Also, being so deathly sick, I wasn't sure that I could go on like this. What a relief that I didn't have to face any more of that awfulness. Think of the worst stomach flu you've ever had, and then multiply that by nine. Days. Weeks. MONTHS. Is it any wonder that I could not comprehend the feeling of being pregnant, much less entertain romantic, dreamy feelings of the child growing within me?!

I'll never forget the distinct peace that came through prayer that night. I was equally at peace with the thought of losing the baby as I was with the thought of actually having one. The sickness had given me a reality check of sorts (although I still had no inkling of how bad it was going to get), and I felt overwhelmed at the thought of how I could get through the pregnancy.

At this point, though, there was nothing to do but wait and let the effects of a miscarriage take their toll through the night. The nurses promised more blood work in the morning and then left us to try to rest.

6 – Six Weeks Along...Or Four Months?

Next morning, the promised blood work was performed, and the results came back rather quickly. My doctor came in to give us the news...again.

"Your numbers are still climbing. In fact, the blood tests show that your hormone levels are that of a pregnant woman who is 4 months along."

We couldn't believe it. I was only six weeks pregnant.

Two things suddenly dawned on me.

"So I *am* pregnant." and "So *that's* why I've been so sick!"

Aloud I said, "So what was causing the pain?" (It had decreased significantly through the night).

"A cyst," said the doctor. "It happens sometimes in pregnancy." He was right, and it eventually took care of itself.

When the week of observation was over, I got to go home. I was so happy to be free, and I left feeling confident of better days ahead. After all, I had a purse full of Gravol and a handful of antacids!

Once at home, I continued to have rough days. Sprinkled among the bad days were a few good ones. By good, I mean that I was able to leave the bed and sit on the couch. It seemed like the Gravol wasn't working as well as it did at first, and it always left me with such horrible headaches and a feeling of dizziness. On good days I was doing good to be able to get out of bed by noon. I would get up, nibble on some toast, and head back to bed. I was so weak that just that hour out of bed completely exhausted me for the rest of the day and evening. A hot shower weakened me even more. My journal entry for December 7, simply says, *"Cooked a meal!"* And the entry for December 19, says, *"Made pancakes!"* Those two food-related accomplishments really were milestones worth recording. I have no clue what my husband ate most of those days. He can't cook, so I'm imagining a lot of cereal and tomato soup was on the table those days. He kept saying he didn't want to eat if I couldn't, and although he did go some days without eating, I think he finally realized that he was going to starve if he waited for me to be hungry!

Our church Christmas cantata was planned for December 18, and guess who was the pianist? I worried a lot about how I was going to get through it. The day came, and I was quite sick; I missed the morning services. By afternoon I was sitting at the kitchen table trying to swallow just a few bites of canned pear so that my stomach wouldn't be empty. I managed to make it to the cantata, armed with plans of what to do if I couldn't make it through. My husband put a snack behind the music rack on the piano. One lady told me later that she was looking around for something I could use if I got sick. She spotted the glass 'vase' being used for decorations on the piano. The only problem? The tube was open ended on both sides. Thankfully, I didn't need it in the end. Looking back, I'm amazed that I got through it. I have no doubt that God was giving me the grace and strength to get through the evening's events, moment by moment.

7 – There's No Place Like Hospital

On December 22, I found myself once again in the emergency room. I had been through several weeks of "getting by" when it comes to eating and drinking (literally surviving on "bird bites"), but the last three days had been brutal. The Gravol, which really only ever brought momentary relief, had completely stopped working. Crystallized ginger no longer soothed my tummy, neither did a long list of other "tried and true" morning sickness cures, including peppermint tea, crackers, canned fruit, banana, toast, mints, lemon water, etc. Liquids bounced when I tried to drink. And I was becoming an expert at learning what foods were the easiest to not keep down. (You know what I mean.) One of the hardest parts was the insatiable thirst and craving I had for fruit and liquids. I remember my intense longing to be able to drink a full glass of cold water! I still remember that mad craving feeling—only it wasn't for watermelon or pickle milkshakes. I just wanted water. That in itself should have been a clue to how dehydrated I really was. But I *didn't* know.

I should share a bit of explanation as to why I was so naive about pregnancy. We lived on an island and most of the people we knew were older. *We* were the youngest people we knew! Most of the women I had contact with had had their babies years ago. We were 2,000 miles from home and family, and I was much too sick to do research online or read books...or call my Mom. My husband, being a relatively new husband, didn't have a clue about morning sickness either. For some reason we both thought that "this is the way it's supposed to be." Not until after the pregnancy did I stop and realize that most women continue on with relatively normal lives while pregnant. They still work, exercise, shop, take care of their other kids, etc., etc. They *don't* live in bed and they *do* eat and drink...enough for two, I might add! They are able to stand up for more than a few minutes and they *don't* make their husbands sleep on the floor for weeks and months on end. Somewhere along the line, it dawned on me that what I had experienced wasn't normal. Gradually, after the birth of our son, I realized just how clueless I had been. Thankfully, I walked into my second pregnancy with eyes wide open, armed with a proactive plan, several HG support sites, and a more knowledgeable husband. (Yes, I had a second pregnancy even after all this!)

Back to the first pregnancy, though. On this particular cold December day, the ER nurses remembered me, which meant less time spent in triage. Realizing that I could barely walk, they gave me a stretcher and an IV a few hours sooner than the previous time. I remember lying there in the ER, when suddenly a paper was being flashed in my face.

"Here, sign this. I cannot do anything for you until you sign this!" I struggled to understand the accent of the man standing in front of my face.

Through the intense nausea, I cracked my eyes open, wondering who was barking at me like that. It was the doctor on call, but he was dressed more like a hippie on call. His long flowing hair was tied back in a ponytail and a bandana was wrapped around his head in biker style. I must not have responded fast enough, because all of a sudden he was waving that paper again, this time with a pen in the other hand. He laid it on my pillow and demanded again that I sign it. I didn't have a clue what the paper said, and being too sick to open my mouth, I didn't even ask.

"She can't even sit up," I heard my husband say, "Can I sign it for her?"

"No, it has to be signed by the patient!" barked the doctor.

I'm pretty sure I signed it with my left hand so I wouldn't have to sit up. It wasn't even legible, but it seemed to appease the doctor. I found out later that he had found out we were from the States, and the paper, if signed, protected him against a patient suing him for any medical decisions he made that might go wrong.

Along with seeing the doctor on call every day, the obstetrician I had seen during my last hospital stay became my specialist for the rest of the pregnancy. I guess it was obvious to them that this girl was going to keep coming back! I had another ultrasound (that was one of the blessings in all this—I got to see the baby a lot!). The baby was a few weeks behind in growth, the amniotic fluid was low, and the baby was very still. But I was only nine weeks and some odd days along, so they figured baby had time to catch up. I spent that night in the outpatient department while they waited for a room to become available. They pushed fluids in me at a pretty fast rate for the first 24 hours. In fact, my IV machine protested having to work so hard. I insisted to my husband that "Mr IV" (pronounced "ivy" in honor of the approaching Christmas season) was talking to me all night. Every few seconds, it sounded like it said, "throw up" in that mechanical, growling way. If you've had an IV a few times or more, you know what I mean. It seemed that ever after that, each IV had a different "phrase" or "song" to offer. We started to see a pattern in this IV thing, so we named each one according to its "personality."

The next morning, Mr. IV came with me to the maternity floor once again. The nurses there remembered me also and welcomed me with "she's back!" in a sing-song voice. I was truly thankful for them—some of them had become friends to us during my last stay, and it was less terrifying to be in the hospital knowing I had friends there.

8 – Christmas At Hospital

On Saturday, Christmas Eve, the on call doctor I had seen in the ER came in with "good news."

"We ought get you home by 'Ho-Ho Day,'" he said.

I was confused. I had only been stabilized for about 24 hours and was not yet allowed to have solid food. My meals consisted of salty broth, juice, and tea or coffee (which I didn't drink). A dietician had come in and figured out what I could and could not have based on my non-diagnosis (I still had not been diagnosed at this point, neither had I even heard of Hyperemesis Gravidarum). My husband would sneak in crackers and canned fruit from the vending machines and I would nibble on those to help my stomach settle. If I heard footsteps approaching my room, I hid the food under my sheets. If they found me with it, they would take it away. It seemed that once I was stabilized, I had to have something more solid or I would get sick from not having food in my stomach—what a crazy cycle! "Should I risk eating, or not? Will it make me feel better, or worse?" was always the question in my mind.

Added to the complication of food was the "minor" detail that I was not able to take any meds by mouth—how then could I survive at home? I remember distinctly not wanting to go home—I knew I would just have to turn around and come back and start the admitting process all over again. I couldn't believe that I actually wanted to stay.

That evening a barbershop quartet came around and sang in our ward. To this day, Jonathan and I agree that we have never heard such beautiful music as we heard that night.

"Silent Night...sleep in heavenly peace."

"Joy to the world...and heaven and nature sing."

The music was like a huge meal to a starved person. We soaked up the first song. Then Jonathan opened our curtain and door so we could see them and they us. They came closer and sang a piece just for us.

"There's a song in the air...for the manger of Bethlehem cradles a King!"

Our hearts felt so blessed! Now every Christmas I think of those who are in the hospital. And I understand how very much it means to just have a visit or a song on a special day, or any day for that matter. It's like a peek into the world that we are missing while being hospitalized.

Sunday was Christmas day. But it wasn't just any Christmas day.

It was our first Christmas together as a married couple.

At home, our Christmas tree was drying out and the gifts underneath were growing impatient. We had had all kinds of plans of how to celebrate together. As a new bride, I carried in my heart the plans of new family traditions we wanted to start. But it seemed as if the only tradition we could get started was being in the hospital together! I'll admit that we were pretty discouraged and lonely. No one called or came to visit, and for a while we had a pity party (without food, of course!).

To make matters worse, my vein collapsed and the IV fluids started flowing freely into my arm. By evening, my arm, aside from being sore, was looking angry and red. You guessed it—Mr. IV had to go and another one was put in. It was a bit less painful going in since I was more hydrated (those things are PAINful going in when you are dehydrated!). My husband is squeamish about needles, so the nurse enlisted the help of Jacob again. He offered his services if I needed to squeeze his hand. He might possibly still be sore from that night!

Most of the week after Christmas was spent with doctors trying different medications, first through IV. I don't even remember all the names of the meds I tried; I just remember that none of them worked. I was still quite sick even while in the hospital, and the mismatch of medications made me feel even worse. One morning they tried one called Stemetil, and I had such a bad reaction to it that I couldn't forget the name of it! It made my whole body feel incredibly sluggish to the point where I couldn't process or follow simple commands. It literally felt like I was outside of my body hearing and seeing things but having no control. It took several hours for that one to wear off, and I was pretty scared to try any more! Being from the United States, I had no idea what medications to ask for; but looking back, I wonder why my specialist didn't try some more well-known medications for nausea, before he broke out his list of "shots in the dark."

One of my doctor's last attempts to control my sickness was to give me a shot of steroids. I remember thinking how strange that was, knowing that steroids are used generally for preemies to speed up lung development. Did he think the baby was going to come alarmingly early? Either way, the shot did nothing to ease the nausea. Furthermore, I broke out in little sores all over my body as a side effect from the shot. Once again, the adverse effects of a medication had to be counter-acted. And I added another medication to my "do not give" list.

Have you ever been so physically weak that you couldn't cry? That was me at this point; I was so overwhelmed, but yet too sick to express it. I remember just sobbing in my heart, even while lying perfectly still, trying not to get sick. The combination of being in a new country, a new culture, having no family around, and having a sickness that no one seemed to know what to do with, all culminated in my heart at once.

I whispered to my husband, "I'm crying in my heart," to which he responded, "I know. I am too."

9 – "You Are Beautiful People"

On Tuesday afternoon, a nurse came in and announced that a psychiatrist was coming in to see me.

"Why?" I asked.

She replied with a nebulous answer that he had been called in to see my husband and myself. We put two and two together and realized that my specialist had probably ordered the referral. Oddly enough, this particular specialist had been hounding me since I had come in about my "need" to go back to the United States to be with my family.

"You are depressed," he would say with his thick accent, "You miss your mom. That is why you are so sick." Of course we thought that was ridiculous! I knew I would be just as sick if my mom were sitting right beside me. But day after day he came in and repeated the same sentiments. He would start by bursting into the door and looking around the room with a frown. Then he would scold us in angry tones, "Why is the shade down?! Open the shade so some light comes in! Why is the TV not on?! Why are you just sitting around doing nothing?!" He threw his hands into the air with disgust.

I was usually feeling too bad to explain that the shades were down because light made my headaches/nausea worse. The TV was not on because we didn't want to spend the money for something we wouldn't watch anyway. We weren't doing anything because...well, there wasn't much to do in the hospital, especially if you can't sit up.

Most days after his visit, I would be in tears and Jonathan would be so mad. The nurses would wait until the doctor was gone, and then they would rush in and apologize for his actions and words. He clearly should not have been working with women. Some months later, when we brought our baby back for an appointment that was in an office next door to his, we noticed that his name was no longer on the sign next to his door. In fact, his nametag had been ripped off the wall with such force that the paint was gone too.

So on this particular day when the psychiatrist came in, I realized that at least one doctor thought we were crazy! We found out later that people thought my husband was abusive and controlling because he was with me almost every minute while I was hospitalized. I was shocked to find out that they viewed his presence this way, knowing that he is the most kind and loving man I know. It seemed so natural to us that we would stay together, especially given the circumstances of being far from home and in a brand new culture. But the culture part was what we didn't understand. Later we came to realize that many husbands and wives lived totally separate lives and often when one spouse or family member was in the hospital, their own family members didn't go to see them, much less stay there with them the entire time. For us, that time in the hospital drew us together and strengthened our marriage. Part of my journal entry from January 3, reads this way:

"...I'm so thankful for my dear husband, who hasn't uttered a single complaint, but has sacrificed his own needs many times to meet mine. Having such a wonderful, loving husband is priceless..."

The psychiatrist greeted us with a smile, which relieved me. But then he insisted that we be separated for interview. I wasn't very happy about that, but was obviously powerless to stop it.

So Jonathan left the room and sat in the waiting area while the psychiatrist evaluated me. For probably 45 minutes he asked me questions related to my health, my immediate family, my upbringing, my husband's character, and my state of contentment in this new country. While I talked, he was busy drawing a detailed graph of what he was hearing. I was pretty confused the whole time, but just tried to calmly answer his questions. When he finished, he thanked me and left. I waited while he talked to Jonathan, and found out later that he had asked the same questions and done the same drawing. I suppose he was trying to make sure our answers lined up with each others'.

After sitting at the nurses' station and completing his notes on us, he arrived back in our room and took a bow (he was foreign).

"You are *beautiful* people!" he beamed, "We so happy to have you in Canada!"

With that, he took another bow, and left the room.

10 – The Ambulance Ride

Tuesday evening, my specialist had mentioned again the possibility of going home. While it sounded nice, I knew that I still was not stable enough to go home and take all of my pills by mouth. Up to this point, I had not even taken prenatal vitamins—it would have been nice just to keep some food down, and then think about taking horse pills! The nurses brought me yogurt and popsicles but they wouldn't stay down either. By Tuesday evening, I was able to keep some soup down, which was progress. We figured out that the hospital cafeteria served really yummy soups every day, and so Jonathan would go down every lunch and supper and bring me a bowl of whatever they were serving. After a few bites, I was finished and he would eat the rest. Many, many meals in the hospital found my tray untouched. And it was all I could do not to get sick when my roommate opened her tray. Hospital food is bad enough without smelling someone else's!

Wednesday morning dawned and our specialist entered our room mid-morning in his usual thunderous style.

"You are going to Halifax," he said, "I cannot do anything else for you."

We were shocked! So it was to be Halifax instead of home. And he was giving up on me?! I had been in this hospital for a week and the doctors really hadn't found what worked; they only seemed to be able to find what didn't work. The mention of "IWK" was reassuring in terms of hospitals. But now, we were going further into the unknown, and farther from home.

The doctor matter-of-factly explained that I would be transferred to IWK by ambulance in about an hour. And what an interesting ride it turned out to be!

The two young men responsible for my transfer were very nice. I wasn't a happy camper when I found out that I had to be on my back for the entire three-hour drive. It is absolute torture for me to be on my back when I'm nauseated. We hit a compromise and he propped me up slightly and I turned a little toward one side. A new, temporary IV was with me at this point and I can't remember its name, but it was responsible for keeping me hydrated until we reached the hospital.

One of the funniest memories we have from that time in our lives happened on the ambulance ride. Somehow, in the transfer of patients, the EMTs had forgotten to re-stock the ambulance. And what should they forget to pack...but the bedpan! I mentioned before that I was on large amounts of continuous fluids...so you get the picture. Halfway through our ride, I needed to use the washroom and could not wait. Actually, my husband needed a washroom too. The EMT dug around for the bedpan, but it just wouldn't turn up. He finally admitted to us (with many apologies) that the ambulance had not been properly restocked before departure. All he had was an extra IV bag, which we were, at this point, happy to see! So they pulled over for a washroom break. We were just that desperate!

11 - HG School

When we arrived at the IWK in Halifax, I was taken up to my new room to get settled in. We were glad to finally get a private room. It had a wonderful view of the city, and the helicopter pad was right above us. The nurses were so friendly and professional, and as soon as the papers were filled out, I was handed a menu.

"Just circle what you want to eat for each meal," the nurse said cheerfully, "And if you don't like what's on the menu, just write in what you'd like to have and they'll make it for you."

Really? Wow, this was quite a change from the last hospital! No more trays of smelly fish (I normally love fish, but I had to wonder if hospital fish ever saw the ocean!) and salty broth. I ordered mac and cheese, fresh fruit, muffins, grilled cheese, salad, and more. I knew I would only be able to eat a few bites at each meal, but it sure felt good to dream about what I thought I might be able to eat. No worries anyway, as my happy husband was the recipient of my leftovers.

Early the next morning, I was awakened by a nurse who obviously didn't check my chart to find out why I was there. She flipped on the light and said it was time to go across the hall to be weighed. I groggily asked her to repeat what she said, to which she gave the same response. I really could not believe that they would rouse a pregnant and very morning-sick lady just to be weighed in. Seriously, I had lost so much weight that I was mere skin and bones. I didn't want to be reminded! Nevertheless, I staggered across the hall into a room with a scale, dizzy and trying not to lose the breakfast I hadn't had yet. Why that weight was so important to get at that moment, I'll never know. But I made sure my nurse put it on my chart not to do that again.

"Could we possibly do that a little later in the day?" I reasoned. She heartily agreed.

During one of the days of my week-long stay at IWK, my nurse came in with a pill called Diclectin. Instead of the trial and error I had experienced before, it seemed like my doctor here had a specific plan for treatment. In fact, he even knew what was wrong with me and he didn't label it as mental! Here at IWK was where I first heard the term *Hyperemesis Gravidarum.*

"Hyper-wha-a?" I asked.

"Hyperemesis Gravidarum," replied the doctor, as if it were the most common condition ever. "It's a pregnancy condition where the woman gets severely sick and dehydrated. Most women who have this need constant medication to control the symptoms. It usually lasts until she gives birth."

Two things hit home for me. The first was that, "my condition has a name!" And the second was that, "this is going to last until I give birth?!" That really was not news I wanted to hear, considering I was only ten weeks and some days along. I surely hoped that they could get this under control very soon so we could assume some sort of a normal life. Using hindsight, I realize that I should have written the term for HG down and taken it home to research more about it. But I promptly forgot the name of it, thinking that finally I would get something that would get it under control for good. It wasn't until our baby was about five months old that I saw and remembered the term again. (More about that later).

The Diclectin took the edge off of the nausea, but didn't take it away enough for me to eat and drink. I was still nibbling throughout the day and sipping ice cold drinks. Coupled with the IV, I was stabilized enough to sit up for a few minutes and have small conversations with people. My husband soon learned that if I got real quiet and stopped saying a few words here and there, I was dealing with the heavy nausea again. If a nurse asked a question and I didn't answer, he would answer for me and tell them why. Most days were up and down, concerning how I felt, but it become increasingly clear that even the Diclectin (which is specially designed for nausea in pregnancy) wasn't helping me function well enough to go home.

12 – The Miracle Drug

Enter Zofran, that wonderful-but-not-designed-for-pregnancy-drug. My nurse brought me a tiny pill one afternoon when I was still complaining of intense nausea. The pill was soft and white. It dissolved under my tongue and it tasted horrible. It was so bitter that it threatened to turn my mouth inside out. But not even minutes after I took the little thing, my nausea just started to melt away. I could almost feel it happening. I couldn't believe how good I felt—the best I'd felt in two and a half months. What was that stuff?!

"Well, it's really a drug for chemo patients," said my nurse, "But we use it sometimes for extreme cases like yours."

"Ok, so now I'm taking drugs that cancer patients use," I thought, "What's going to be next?"

The nurse went on to tell me that I would not be able to have Zofran very often—it was just there to use sparingly. That made me a bit frustrated, although I understood that they had good reasons. We had finally found what worked and I wasn't going to be allowed to have it very much. To this day, I still call it the miracle drug. And little did I know that in the weeks ahead I would end up needing it (and getting it) around the clock.

I decided to enjoy those short 4-6 hours I would have as a somewhat normal feeling person. I actually got out of bed and took a short walk around the hall with my husband and IV. We sat in the patient lounge and watched the helicopters coming and going with patients. We watched the goings-on in the city. And we ate! For the first time in almost three weeks, I ate a regular meal. I went crazy asking for whatever I could think of that was yummy to eat—jello, fruit, breads, yogurt, ham, veggies, etc. It was so weird to feel actually hungry and to know that the food would stay down. Jonathan went crazy eating too, since he had been skimping a lot on meals while I was sick. We even squirreled our leftovers away for the next morning, anticipating a large appetite at breakfast time.

Of course, by evening the Zofran had worn off, and the squirreled leftovers went uneaten the next day. But it was fun to dream!

13 – "Grow Our Baby...Nothing Else Matters"

We rang in the new year of 2006 with as little celebration as our first Christmas had held. We could hear the fireworks in the city, but we couldn't see them from our room or the patient waiting room. The first part of my journal entry on January 3, reads:

"Another year gone, another year ahead; but it seems like just a blurry addition to the old one."

Time has a way of becoming intangible when one spends concentrated amounts of time doing the same thing. Many, many uninterrupted hours, days, and weeks were spent with me concentrating on not getting sick. I couldn't even feel time anymore. It felt like we were in the middle of a nightmare that had no end and no beginning. I had forgotten what it was like to feel good. And I couldn't even imagine eating three full meals per day. Another dream that eluded me was the glorious pleasure of gulping down cool liquids. Even though I wanted to do it so badly, the thought of opening my mouth to drink was nauseating. It took effort even to sip through a straw.

With Zofran no longer on my list of options, my doctor decided to increase my dosage of Diclectin to three pills per day. That actually gradually helped me become more functional, and I was weaned off the IV.

"This means, though," said my nurse, "that you have to start drinking enough to replenish the fluids you were getting through IV, and you need to start taking prenatal vitamins."

That would definitely be the hard part. But I was so ready to go home that I would have agreed to just about anything!

I was "somewhat" discharged, meaning I was no longer under the constant care of a nurse. I was moved down the hall to a different section of rooms. I still had access to help if I needed it; but if I developed persistent needs, I would have to be re-admitted. Unfortunately, home IV therapy is not an option in the maritime area where we lived and received treatment, so this room was where the trial began of whether or not I could make it on my own. Apparently, I did well enough to satisfy the doctor, and I was soon released to go home!

After we packed up to leave, we both had a realization: We had come to the hospital in an ambulance. How were we supposed to get home? Jonathan got on the phone and began calling around to price our options. Taking a bus was out of the question—the three-hour drive home was quoted at an exorbitant amount! Taking a taxi was even more out of the question because of cost. It looked like renting a car was our only option. So we booked a car, and they brought it to the hospital to pick us up. Then we drove back to the rental company to sign the papers. I know we must have been a sight to behold—we hadn't known we were coming to Halifax, much less that we would be in two hospitals for almost three weeks. I know I had my pillow and a few changes of clothes. Jonathan must have had at least one change of clothes with him, but that was all. I remember many days when he showered and put the same clothes right back on. There really wasn't any other option.

We put our few belongings in the car and drove to a department store to load up on electrolyte drinks and juice. We also bought a humidifier at the recommendation of our doctor. He seemed to think that moist air would help me feel better. I'm pretty sure he was grasping at a straw for that one, but at that point we were trying anything that the doctors and nurses thought would help. We also got my prescription for Diclectin filled—enough for one month. I felt like we were on the home stretch. Normalcy was on its way.

When we finally arrived home, I had been in two hospitals for three weeks. It felt like three years.

Upon opening our front door and stepping inside, we found our Christmas tree browned over. Completely dead.

I touched the tree with one finger. In the silence of our cold and neglected living room, a shower of needles hit the gifts underneath and then scattered on the hardwood floor.

So symbolic. So heart wrenching. Yet so reassuring....so hopeful. I had survived, once again, what doctors said I may not survive. I was home, at least for that day.

Christmas wasn't a place. It wasn't a tradition. It wasn't even the dream of what I wanted it to be.

It was our hearts. It was Christ. It was God's will, which was bigger than my dreams of the perfect Christmas.

My journal entry from January 3, (the day we got home from the hospital) reads:

"We spent our first Christmas together in the hospital. It was hard not to be home, but many others were there also. We learned that we had the most precious gifts right there with us—Jesus our Savior, each other, and our growing baby.

We welcomed 2006 in a hospital room, but hopefully the lessons and patience learned will follow throughout life. Goals for this year? Grow our baby, love my husband more, serve and know God better. Nothing else matters."

14 – New of the Same

Chicken pox are bad enough when you get them as a child. Thankfully, I had them then. My husband didn't. My journal entry for January 22, says this:

"From bad to worse. Now Jonathan has chicken pox! I am not a very good nurse."

Poor fellow! And poor me. When I finally got up in the late afternoons, I couldn't even look at him. I definitely couldn't eat anything around him. I did my best to make him oatmeal baths and paint calamine lotion on him until I was nauseated again. He had a really bad case of them, complete with a high fever and pox in his throat. He still has scars from that experience. Maybe I do too?!

After the pox episode passed, our version of normal life resumed. It was new days of the same, really. By late January, I had passed the supposedly magical 3-month mark—yet the sickness continued. I learned quickly to cherish any good moments that I had. When I felt good for several hours straight—what relief! It seemed I was a new person, and I began to take advantage of those times. If only it would last! Going out had begun to be difficult, as any good moment could change instantly and begin the sickness cycle. I was afraid to go to the grocery store (and definitely not alone!) or anywhere that didn't have a washroom that was instantly accessible. A place to lie down was an added bonus... (why don't they have those in stores?!)

My journal tells me that I did actually venture out of hiding one winter day:

January 24 - *"First time out of the house in 3 weeks. I found some baby clothes on sale."* I still remember that outing.

I went with some ladies from church to the grocery store and to a little second-hand shop, where I bought a tiny dress. It was the first time I had been in town since getting home from the hospital. Once home, it had been three more rough weeks at home before I had the strength to go out. I felt like a stranger who had been in hiding—almost like I was a strange life form who didn't belong out in public! But it sure was good therapy and the fresh, cold air felt good on my face.

January of that year also marked the happy fact that we had been married for eight months. In doing some quick math, I realized that three of those months had been spent in and out of hospitals together. I felt rotten at the way our new marriage was going. No, we weren't having "marriage troubles" but once again expectations had sabotaged my thinking of what our first year was going to be like. Guilt often crept into my heart. I was supposed to be a shining example of the perfect new wife, and most days I couldn't even lift my head up from my pillow. Forget cooking meals and cleaning the house. Reality had set in for Husband as well—he was on his own!

15 - HG Lifestyle

I mentioned earlier that HG is life altering; the severity varies depending on the woman and the different influencing factors in her life. But exactly what was our HG lifestyle like? I'm going to let you peek into my journal again to get a glimpse of how things were. Also I want to tactfully give you an idea of what the physical symptoms were like.

January 30 - *"15 weeks pregnant. Diclectin isn't working anymore. If I can get up briefly by noon or 1 it's a good day."*

So if that was a good day, what was a bad day like? Well, a bad day found me in bed for the whole 24 hours, and invaded the next day too. My husband sat in a chair at the foot of the bed and read to himself. On really bad days, he couldn't even speak or shuffle in his seat without my getting sick instantly. That's how intense the nausea was. When I had an episode of vomiting, he would assist me by pointing the fan directly on me (hot flashes threatened to cause me to faint) and by dashing to put an ice-cold washcloth on my neck. It was the same every time. If he had been out of the room for a while and wanted to re-enter, he would stand at the door and wait for my signal of whether or not I could tolerate his entering the room. I would blink my eyes for "yes" and keep my eyes closed for "no." Morning and evening ran together and I lost all sense of time.

The nausea and sickness aggravated a vicious cycle, and I started missing pills because I just couldn't get them down. Often when I did get them down, they bounced. To complicate matters, I began developing bedsores from lying so tensely in the same position for so many hours at a time. I had lost so much weight so quickly that my bones were protruding through a very thin skin layer. My whole body was so incredibly sore! I still remember vividly that pain; often it was almost as intense as the nausea was, and relief for the pain would have only come through getting up and moving around, which I couldn't do much of. So our only solution was to double-fold soft blankets and pile them two or three deep to give extra padding. Even that didn't help for the long term, but it was better than just the mattress. I also had to wear special support hose for the entire time I was bedridden, to prevent blood clots from forming since I was so immobile. On good days, I was usually able to take a shower by early evening, with assistance from my husband. Any time I stood up for a length of time, I was in danger of passing out, so my showers and baths were short and always left me utterly exhausted. If I washed my hair, I didn't have the strength to blow dry it. So I would go back to bed and spread my hair out over the pillow. Jonathan would finish the job by blow drying it and brushing it out, then pulling it back into a loose ponytail.

Beside our bed was sleeping bag and a pillow—Jonathan's bed for about six months of the pregnancy. Thankfully, he is the type who can sleep pretty much anywhere! He wanted to be close by in case I needed him (I was so weak that I couldn't talk loud) so the living room couch was too far away. I was usually able to get about five hours of sleep per night. Often the nausea lessened by late evening, allowing for a few hours of rest before my body awoke at 5:00 AM or earlier and the cycle had begun for another day. I would set the alarm for midnight and take my medicine, hoping it would work through the night and ease the nausea I had upon waking. Sometimes it worked, and sometimes it didn't.

HG is very unpredictable, and does not like to follow patterns. A food that stayed down one day might not be tolerable the next day. So there was no use in stocking up on a newly found "miracle food" since it would become less-than-miraculous by a day or two later. And of course the usual intolerance of food smells was part of my life. If Jonathan decided to cook something, he had to first close my bedroom door, then open some windows before starting to heat something up. It was usually something simple like tomato soup, toast, or eggs. HG took us by surprise, so I had no time to teach him how to cook. He learned by trial and error!

Also included in the lifestyle of HG are "flare-ups." Flare-ups usually happened after I had exerted myself physically above normal. Some days "above normal" consisted of simply sitting up or taking a shower. Other days we had to make the 2- hour plus round trip off the island and to the hospital for an appointment, and it was fairly predictable that the next day would find me violently ill. I was amazed at how quickly I lost weight and at how weak I became after just days in bed. But considering the fact that my body was running on zero fuel, it makes sense. A flare-up was characterized by non-stop vomiting and debilitating nausea. I know, I said that's what my normal days were like! They were, but a flare-up took the violence of the symptoms to another level. Usually when I ended up in the hospital again, it was the result of a flare-up. My specialist repeatedly blamed these occurrences on food poisoning. We knew, of course, that that wasn't the case, as I wasn't even eating more than "bird bites" of fruit, much less undercooked or restaurant food that could have made me sick.

Part of our HG lifestyle was music, mostly traditional, instrumental hymns. My husband would put a CD into the player each morning, and that was my day's music. I counted the hours by how many times the CD repeated itself. The volume was kept very low so as not to jar my senses and make me sicker. I concentrated on the music so hard that I knew the playlist order, and how each song started and ended. I even memorized the flow of the songs, anticipating the specific musical identities of each arrangement. To this day, I still cannot listen to some of those CDs without having vivid memories with each song. Truthfully, I still own them but I can't bring myself to play them. To change things up a bit during my second pregnancy, I ordered some CDs that have Scripture being read with instrumental music in the background. And I bought a special CD to use during labor. I saved it until "birth day" so that it wouldn't have bad memories associated with it. The music I listened to during HG was my lifesaver in a way; it helped give me something to concentrate on besides trying not to get sick. And as I tried to focus on the words of the arrangements I was hearing, it brought a measure of peace to my heart to know that God was still in control. While there were many times when my faith waned, the reinforcement of Scripture and song helped me keep my head above water spiritually.

I missed many weeks of church services, and on the days when I tried to make it to a service, it literally took me hours to get up, shower, and dress. By then I was exhausted, and sometimes I ended up right back in bed. A few times I pushed myself to go anyway, only to have to leave just in time to get sick. My journal records the few times I was able to make it to church with phrases like *"Got to go to church!"* or *"Made it to both services!"* It really was a big deal to get up and dressed and be able to sit in church. We were blessed that the church was literally steps away from the parsonage and didn't involve car travel.

Hindsight, I have some regrets. If I had it to do over, I wouldn't pressure myself so much to go to church and other events. I would try to be more content with resting, and entertain fewer thoughts of "what I should be doing." When you practically give your life up to grow your child, it brings a different perspective to all of life.

16 – Flutters and Feelings

February 1st records perhaps the first "normal" part of my pregnancy: *"Felt baby 'flutter' for the first time."* The first flutter felt like a tiny vibration in my tummy—short and intermittent, but with a distinct pattern. It took me awhile to even realize what the feeling was. I was fifteen weeks and a few days along, still thin and tiny. No baby pooch here, but now I had a definite sign of life. So far, it had felt like fifteen weeks of the worst stomach flu ever. I spent a lot of time just trying to convince myself that there was a baby inside, hoping that the "mushy" feelings would come and I would be able to cope with my condition better. It didn't work. All of the "new mommy" feelings I had heard about were evading me.

Let's take a moment, shall we, and talk about feelings? The weeks between fifteen and twenty of the pregnancy were the crisis point for me. Not only did I reach my lowest physically, but I hit rock bottom emotionally. The severity of the symptoms and the constancy of the suffering without relief did their work on me. Many were the times that I was too weak to cry physically, but inside my heart was sobbing great heaving sobs of grief. I tried so *hard* to want this. But being unable to even comprehend the presence of a child within me, I often secretly wished for it to slip up to heaven. We would both be better off. After all, baby wasn't getting any nourishment. The common cliché that "babies always get what they need" is a serious fallacy for HG patients. If the mother is not taking in nutrients for days on end, then there is nothing for the baby to receive. Yes, it saps some of the reserve of the mother (if there is any), but that in turn leaves the mother weaker.

Perhaps my dehydrated brain did not process things rightly during this time. I suffered often from splitting headaches as a result of the combination of dehydration and the continual violence of my sick episodes. All I could do was lay there and beg prayers—heart prayers that seemed unanswered all.

The result? Wishing for a miscarriage. As hard as that is to admit, it is truth. And if you've ever been in a seriously ill and confused position where there seemed no hope and doctors shook their heads, perhaps you can understand. My heart wanted the suffering to end for both myself and the baby. I wanted time—more time to research and to prepare. More time to be a wife. More time to wrap my head around if and how I could do this mother thing. *"Why is it so hard for me?"* I often wondered. *"Most women I know WORK almost the entire pregnancy. How on earth do they do it?"* In the fog of illness, lack of experience, and the absence of young women to socialize with, I honestly thought that everyone was this sick, but somehow they managed to keep going. Was I ever naïve! Thinking I would soon be better after Christmas, I had forgotten the name of the disease I heard about in Halifax hospital, nor did I have the resources or ability to do my own research at the time. "So this is morning sickness," I thought.

17 – Something Special

On February 2, we received a box in the mail. We were overjoyed, since we didn't often get "real" mail from the States. I opened a box from my Grandmama and my hands fell onto two afghans and some crocheted baby footies. So soft and pretty...I knew that she had handmade them, as was her custom of showing love to her family. These items were the first baby accessories we received, aside from the little dress I had picked up at the second-hand shop. I treasure these handmade items even more now, since my Grandmama went to heaven recently.

Journal entry from February 10, says,

"Tonight we asked God to do something special for us. We've been kind of down with everything going

wrong...me being so sick and no medicine working, no car (we were borrowing a car since our own car was waiting to be imported into Canada), etc. We just need a token for good!"

February 11 brought our prayed-for token for good: "Today we got our 'something special.' I started the day throwing up, as usual. We prayed, as usual, but this time God saw fit to make me feel better. So I got up and had a nice day. Thank you, LORD!"

Valentine's Day dawned and I felt well again. We actually left the house and went to a restaurant. It was a big deal. I remember being pretty nervous. I worried that any moment I would begin to feel sick and we'd have to leave. But I made it through and we had a lovely time. It felt good to be around civilization!

Shortly after this date, Jonathan felt the baby move for the first time. It was slowly starting to feel real. At eighteen weeks pregnant, I still wasn't showing at all. In fact, I weighed less than ever. But there was life in there, and now my husband could share the experience.

18 – Mounting Bills and Pressure to Abort

Just a few days after our date, I had a doctor's appointment with my gynecologist. It meant making the long trip to the town where the hospital was...again. Doc was not a very pleasant or positive fellow, and often asked us questions we couldn't really answer. In his thick, African accent he shouted and waved his arms, "Why don't you just move back to the States...nothing goes right for you!" And, when he found out that we didn't have medical coverage, he wanted to know "why do you not ask the church for more money?! You do not get what you do not ask for! You have no money, no car, no family!" I think he really thought we were crazy. My husband tried to explain that we were in ministry, but it served only to deepen his cynical thoughts.

Repeatedly he pushed us to have an abortion. He also pushed us to get the genetic testing, stating that it was likely that the baby would have problems due to my prolonged illness. We are not against genetic testing, but at that point, it would have just meant another test to go through. Also, we assured him that the test results would make no difference to us. We were keeping our baby—it was in God's hands.

I left his office in tears every single time we went. Instead of fighting with me for my baby's life, he made me feel guilty for being sick and tried to push for my baby's death. *"How can the same doctor that is supposed to be taking care of me be trying to end my baby's life?"* I wailed to my patient, listening husband.

One such visit to this doctor found us with renewed mental strength, wherein we insisted that he never speak to us again about abortion. We tried many times to speak of Christ to this man, but it was rocky ground. He was a Hindu, so one day we gave him a copy of a book that tells the story of a Hindu who accepted Christ. Doc seemed genuinely thankful to receive the book, and we prayed once again for his eyes to be opened to the truth. *"Maybe, just maybe, God is allowing me to be so sick so we can minister to this man."*

On this particular February day (the 22nd), he changed my medicine again. This time the med carried risks with it because of my history with epilepsy and seizures. It was a tough decision whether or not to use it, but we decided that we would at least give it a try. Doc made us sign a form stating that we would not sue him if I had a serious reaction to the medication or if my seizures returned.

We left his office and went upstairs to get blood work done. It cost $240. My journal entry for that day records our dilemma, *"Ahhh! We are so in debt that it's not even believable! About $35,000 we owe so far. Yep. Then to have to pay for blood work and medicine..."*

Tears bathed our pathway home and we cried out to God for relief in many areas of our life. What on earth was He doing?

19 – "Please Let Me Die"

Oh, how quickly the tide can turn...and February 24, proved that. A flare-up began, and escalated to the point where we knew we were going to have to return to the hospital. Looking back, I stayed home way too long because I dreaded so much going back to the hospital. Also, we didn't know the definite signs of dehydration. Boy, do I know now!

I threw up for 30 hours straight, about every hour at first. The longer it went on, the time in between episodes began to get shorter until I was sick every 20-30 minutes. Pure acid was all that was in my tummy, and I've never had burning like that in my life. Even after I eventually got rehydrated at the hospital, my throat and esophagus were sore for days—they literally had deep burns from my illness.

During those awful hours, my husband prayed aloud for me, begging God to ease my suffering so that we wouldn't have to make the long trip to the hospital. In my weak state, I begged the same from within my heart.

Evening was coming on, and we were deciding whether or not we should go in. Such a no-brainer, but this first time mom didn't know *anything*. I found out later at the hospital that I had lost seventeen pounds in that 30-hour period. I was now in the low 90s and plunging ever lower in my weight.

A knock came on the door. It was a lady from the church. She came and knelt at my side and cried for me. She told us we needed to go in, and right away. She stayed for a few minutes and chatted, then handed Jonathan an envelope and left. He opened it and found $100 in it. Only God knows how much we needed that money. It wasn't just the fact of needing money...He knew we would need cash for our next hospital stay. Parking wasn't free, and neither was food or any of the other myriad of needs that arise when one is hospitalized. What a blessing that card was to us! I still have it—a reminder to me that God cared, even in one of my darkest hours.

Through the night my prayers turned from pleas for healing to *"God, please let me die!"* Oh, how the acid ripped at my throat. And I was so faint that I could barely sit up. Waves of heat rushed over me, taking turns with violent chills that gave my husband the cue to pile the blankets on. A few minutes later he'd have to pull them off again.

When I began bringing up bile and eventually blood, we knew we no longer had a choice. We *had* to go to the emergency room. Jonathan practically carried me to the car, where I slumped in the front seat in my jammies, hair definitely awry. I couldn't have cared any less about my appearance. My whole body was so parched that my tongue was dry and I craved liquids so badly I could cry. My eyes were so dry that it was getting hard to keep them open without pain.

Once to the hospital, Jonathan got a wheelchair and brought me right into the nurse's office. I told her I needed to lie down right away. Surprisingly, she obliged. I have literally lain on the waiting room floor so many times while waiting long hours to be seen. This time I think she took one look and knew I needed to lie down immediately.

No waiting this time—they brought an IV and began the long process of getting it into my arm. Most of the "beautiful veins" in my arms had collapsed and my skin was dry and tight. They resorted to using a baby needle, and decided to put the IV in the back of my hand (one of the most painful spots). The pain was excruciating, and then almost instantly I could feel the cold liquid rushing into my veins. I could tell by the sound of the IV pump that the liquid was being pushed through as fast as the machine was capable of—faster than ever before. *Swirrr, click. Swirr, click. Swirr, click.* Oh, how good it felt! And how I longed to have some of it on my tongue.

During her routine checks, the nurse shined her light into my eyes. She sighed and shook her head. "If you had waited any longer," she said with her eyebrows raised, "You wouldn't have made it."

Just as quickly as the IV went in, I received nausea meds. My husband read the label on the bag. It was Zofran! The miracle drug had returned. In a matter of about fifteen minutes, I began to feel better. Nausea ebbed away, and I felt human. I was allowed to have ice chips (those *wonderful* little squares!). They soothed my raw throat and life became a bit more bearable. I knew I would be admitted soon, and uttered a prayer that they would send me to the maternity floor again. The atmosphere was so much more pleasant on the maternity floor as opposed to the surgical recovery floor or such like, as I had been on other occasions. However, that was not my biggest worry—at least they had a bed for me. There were other times when I stayed on a stretcher in the hallway for hours.

The porter came and my bed was wheeled through hallways, into elevators, and onto an upper floor of the hospital. As soon as I saw the pink walls I knew that my prayer had been answered! I sighed with thanks to God, Who knew how much that meant to me. As we rounded the corner, I saw the familiar faces of nurses who had become friends to me during my many lengthy stays on that floor. They smiled at me and sang out, "She's back!" Yet another reassurance that this was my second home.

As I settled into my room, my thoughts turned to how close I had been to passing away. How could I have not known? Now I worried about my baby. *"If my body was that dry,"* I thought, *"how could the baby possibly be ok?"* I began to be very drowsy, and fell asleep for the first time in over 48 hours.

20 – Anti-Depressants Are the Answer?

Later that evening, a doctor came in to see me. I assumed he was the doctor on call, but I found out later that he wasn't. I was still in a fog as he began firing questions at me:

"So what brought you to Canada?"

"Do you want to be here?"

"Do you ever want to go back to the States?" *(Why does everyone keep asking me that?!)*

"Did your husband force you to come here with him?"

My husband tried to answer for me on some of them, as he could see I was tired and foggy. The doctor shushed him quickly and said that he wanted to hear my answers. I answered weakly, but honestly. I did want to be in Canada, and I didn't want to go back to the States. We were in God's will, and nothing, not even this trial, could convince us to leave! My husband did not force me to come with him—I came willingly.

I thought I did a good job at answering, but I found out later that I must not have. Doc prescribed for me a sleeping pill, one he said, "will help you rest."

"I wasn't having any trouble resting," I thought, *"until you came in and woke me up."*

That night, I awoke in the middle of the night and was once again violently sick. I felt desperately afraid that my new-found miracle drug had lost its affect already. Lack of sleep was taking its toll on me, and I was worn down emotionally. Nurses attended me and we made it through another rough night.

The next evening, my nurse brought me the little plastic cuplet that held a pill. I was to try to take that pill by mouth again, as I had done the night before.

"I don't want the sleeping pill," I said to the nurse.

"What sleeping pill?" she asked.

"The one they gave me last night—I don't want that one again. It made me really sick." Her face was changing as I spoke. She opened her mouth and slowly answered.

"That wasn't a sleeping pill you had. It was an anti-depressant."

Oh, I was angry. My husband was angry. We had not asked for that pill. The doctor had decided that I needed it, and had lied to us, telling us it was a sleeping pill.

"Can you look up the side effects of this medication?" I asked the nurse.

I peeked through my metal blind to the nurses' station and watched her pull out a very thick book and start flipping the pages.

She brought the book to me and let me read the section for myself. "Side effects: nausea, vomiting, etc."

"That's why I'm *here*!" I said desperately to the nurse.

It seemed that we spent a good deal of time fighting the idea that any illness could be traced back to a mental problem. Somehow doctors thought that I was sick because I missed "home" in the States, and that the instant I was placed back in my original environment, I would be miraculously well.

Why were they so reluctant to diagnose Hyperemesis? And why were they so non-proactive about cases like mine? Was I the only one fighting for my life and my baby's?

These questions and more I brought to my pillow that night. It took everything in us not to file an official complaint about that doctor's deception. Some days I still wish that we had, but at the time we didn't want to rock the boat of my care anymore than it was already rocking. We simply let it go. But I never again took a pill without knowing exactly what it was for, what the dosage was (one time I even caught a nurse's mistake on a dose that was too high), and what the side effects were. We were finally learning how to work with the system.

A dietician was called in shortly after my hospitalization to discuss what foods I could tolerate. At the time, I was on an all-liquid diet, and each day that she came in, it was the same story. I couldn't stand even talking about food, much less have the ability to implement what she thought was a good plan for eating. This was another area where we scratched our heads, wondering why the dietician was sent to a patient who couldn't keep anything down. We finally came to realize that a lot of what went on was just protocol. Even common sense could not prevail!

21 – God Has Other Plans

By Sunday in the hospital, I was feeling better, and began to have the strength to get up for a few minutes at a time. I even wrote in my own journal, instead of dictating or writing details down after the fact: *"Answer to prayer—I saw Lisa, a nurse we know who claims to be a Christian. We had a good talk with her. The nurses seem like family now after all of these hospital stays."*

Lisa was one of our favourite nurses. She was the one who held me a few months earlier when we were told that we'd lost our baby. Each time I was hospitalized it seemed she was assigned to me. On this February day we talked about how God's will doesn't always include our ideas of how things ought to go.

"Sometimes God has other plans," she said with a smile. The more I questioned the nurses, the more I realized that I was in for a long haul until this baby was born. Although the nurses were careful and tactful, they let me know gently that my condition was not going to go away. It was time to accept this long-term trial as God's will. My dreams of a happy, normal pregnancy were not reality, nor would they ever be. I grieved that realization. I grieved it for months after Caleb's birth. Yes, even years went by while I held in my heart the grief of why it had to happen that way. *Why me? Why did I have to fall into the 1% of women who suffer with this condition?* HG was a killer of dreams, and I had a lot of things to work through emotionally and spiritually long after the pregnancy ended. In some ways, my second pregnancy had a healing effect on my heart. In other ways, it bore the reality in deeper that nothing would ever be normal. I needed to release my girlhood dreams and embrace God's plan, however nonsensical it seemed at the time.

By putting me in the hospital, God kept us from making a mistake concerning a car that we were about to purchase. A friend from the church had been looking for a vehicle for us, and had recently found one that he recommended. We had committed to giving him an answer on the purchase when we saw him at church Sunday.

Well, that was today and I was trapped in a hospital bed.

My journal comes to our aid again and shines some light on the details of this small event, but one that proved to be significant in the long run:

"We were supposed to give C-- an answer about the car today. We were going to tell him 'yes', and then I ended up in the hospital. But we found out later that the battery is no good and the car has some other problems we didn't know about. So, in a way, God kept us from buying it by putting me in the hospital (I'm sure He has more reasons than that!) And guess what? Now we're paying for my medications and there is NO WAY we could have made payments on the car anyway."

It had been one of those times when God seems very far away...even non-existent. But once in a while, a beam of light broke through and we could see that God really was organizing details in our life—just not the ones we were praying for or expecting.

22 - Truth from a Hindu

On March 1, while still in the hospital, I got to have my fourth ultrasound. This time it was a bit easier to get all of the water down, and I was hoping to see the baby in action. Secretly I wished that this ultrasound would bring some reality to the fact that I was with child, not just suffering from a horrible, non-curable flu!

In some parts of Canada, the doctors are not allowed to tell mothers what they are having. This was the case in our province, and so we didn't even ask when we went in. In fact, sometimes the technician would even turn the screen away and we saw nothing. This time was different, though, and she let me watch.

Although I do not actually remember this particular ultrasound, my journal remembers for me:

"Today I had an ultrasound (my 4th one) and we got to see the baby move. 'He' actually grabbed his foot and brought it to his mouth. 'She' was wiggling so much that the tech couldn't get a very good picture at first. Miraculously, by all measurements the baby is perfectly on track developmentally at 19 ½ weeks. What a blessing!"

After the ultrasound, the technician offered to print off a profile picture of our baby. Then she added that it would cost ten dollars. We turned it down, knowing that we literally did not have that much (that little) to spare. Between owing $35,000 plus the current hospital stay (we didn't have the bills yet), my medications, and parking and food costs for Jonathan during my stay, we were already in over our heads.

Do I regret choosing not to purchase the photo? In some ways, yes. I'm sure the technician thought we were the strangest couple ever. But knowing how things were financially at the time, it really was all we could do. I only have one ultrasound photo of our little girl, for similar reasons. By the time I was pregnant with her, we were paying for my medications, but we had medical coverage for the hospitalizations. Sometimes when I look at Charity's picture, I wish I had one of Caleb to match. But in the grand scheme of things, I know it is not a big deal. There were far more important lessons to be learned during those difficult days. In Caleb's scrapbook, I do have one "womb" item—a printout of contractions and movements during labor. It's pretty special.

On March 3, my doctor came in to my hospital room as usual. We had fulfilled our expected protocol for how he wanted our room to look when he arrived—shades up, me sitting in a chair, etc. On this particular day, he came in with a smile—very unusual! He announced that he was releasing me since I was now stabilized and able to take my medications orally.

The next thing he said shocked and humbled us. "God has been very good to you," came out of the mouth of a Hindu. Wow. He went on to explain how surprised and pleased he was that the baby's growth was on track, considering how sick I had been. We all knew what each other was thinking—that by human standards either me or the baby (or both) shouldn't be here.

Doc's words about God's goodness were a rebuke to me, especially coming from a man who didn't know Christ. Here I had been feeling sorry for myself for being so sick, and *he* was telling *me* how good my God was. Shouldn't it be the other way around?

My journal records a final blessing that occurred literally just before we left the hospital:

"We had to make the decision whether or not to go on Zofran (the chemo drug—the only one that works). It costs about $13-$16 PER PILL, and I'll need 3-4 PER DAY. If you do the math, that's about what my husband makes per week. There is no cheaper generic brand. We prayed, and felt God leading us to do it and to trust Him. Right before we left, my nurse came in and gave me five days' worth of leftover Zofran pills. What a huge blessing! It's scary to think how we are going to afford this medication after today, but we look forward to seeing God provide for us."

The Lord worked His blessings into my heart all the way home as I pondered everything that had happened in the last few months. I was brought to the place of repentance for my attitude and actual gratefulness for God's goodness to our little family.

23 - In Some Way Or Other

You may be familiar with the song, "In some way or other, the LORD will provide."

These weeks following my latest hospitalization were the testing ground for our faith. And, oh, how it was tested! Even our feeble faith was rewarded with God's miracles of provision for his needy sparrows.

One afternoon I received a phone call from a doctor on the mainland who wasn't even my doctor. We lived on an island, in a very small community, and word had gotten back to him that I was now on Zofran.

"Why are you taking that?" he asked, and then proceeded to tell me the dangers of being on that medication while pregnant. It was *not* designed for pregnancy, he said, and it could cause serious harm to the baby. All of these facts he was absolutely correct in stating, and we were already aware of the risks. However, after five months of trial and error, and having just found something that worked, we knew it was the best thing for the present situation. The doctor wasn't too pleased with my reasons and mumbled something about us not being able to afford the medication. I hung up feeling rotten, but knowing there was nothing else we could do.

Just how expensive that medication would be was dawning on us quickly. The amount of pills I needed for one week's time came to the total of $270. My husband was making $300 per week at the time. We had just enough to tithe to our local church, and then go buy my Zofran. Keep in mind that I was on a regimen of four medications and an antacid—all at maxed-out doses. So, after Zofran, there were *three more medications* to buy. I'm really not sure how we bought any groceries. I've asked my husband and he can't remember either. I know we ate a lot of toast and tomato soup.

Aside from my medication costs, the total of my hospital bills now amounted to $50,000, owed to three hospitals and a myriad of doctors. Each hospital and doctor billed separately, so almost daily the mailbox yawned and gave us a new bill to open.

Although we made it a point never to talk about our financial needs, we had to mention the bills when our six-month term at the church was over. It was time for us and the church to decide —should we stay or should we go?

Journal entry for March 12 - *"Discouraging meeting about whether or not we can stay. With all these bills (which now amount to $50,000) they want to know how we plan to make it. Truth be told, we don't know. We're pretty overwhelmed and discouraged. Doesn't seem like God would send us up here, only to send us back, but He could, I guess."*

Meanwhile, we were doing frantic research about some kind of aid to help pay for the Zofran. We found an application online that suggested that we could get some of it free, if signed by a doctor. Jonathan made the long trek to the hospital to see our gynecologist and got the required signature. This was our answer! Or so we thought. We mailed the form in, and received a letter shortly thereafter. Our request had been denied by the company. No explanation was given. Back to square one!

In the weeks that followed, some miraculous things happened. The not-so-miraculous in this scenario was the constant in-pouring of hospital and doctor bills. But then, how could we have a miracle without the need for a miracle? I will admit that we did not always have strong faith in this area. Often the mail came while my husband was at work. I would open the bill(s) and add it to the growing pile of unpaid statements. And often Jonathan would come home and find me sobbing on the couch. A combination of pregnancy hormones and the overwhelming amount of money that we owed merged to make one miserable mama-to-be. I felt guilty that I had caused this financial stress to my husband, the provider for our family.

We began a custom that continued until the culmination of our financial miracle. A basket under the coffee table held the large stack of bills to be paid. Several times a week we took the basket out and laid out all of the bills on the coffee table. We prayed over each one. Well, my husband prayed. I cried while he prayed. There seemed no way out. We tried not to do the math, but how can you not?

When the bills had finally all come in, our total money owed came to $50,000 and some change. Massive debt for a new couple who hadn't even bought a house or car yet, let alone splurged on credit cards. We broke down and did the math. At the rate we were paying ($10 per month), it would take us 120ish years to pay off what we owed. Reality check. God had to do something! We envisioned our child graduating from college while we were still paying off the pregnancy. And long after our children were grown and our grandchildren were grown, they would still be paying off the bills from their Grandmother's pregnancy. Perhaps the humor got us through another tough spot in this season of our lives.

More prayer, and we re-packed the bills into the basket and returned it to its place.

Not only did the paper bills arrive, but soon phone calls began to interrupt our day. I became afraid to answer the phone. The doctors and hospitals called at least once per week, wondering how we planned to pay our bills. Each one billed separately, so that increased the number of calls. My husband began taking care of those calls, since I usually ended up in tears. *Didn't they understand that every penny we got was already going towards my expensive medications, and that we hardly had enough to live on?*

Jonathan promised each caller that we would do our best. Then they began demanding that we commit to paying a certain amount per month. We promised $10. They were not impressed. It was a lot like faith promise, this commitment. We hadn't a clue how, where, or when we would get the money.

And then, a beautiful thing happened. Money started trickling in, bit by bit. We hadn't said a word to people about what we owed. We wanted to see God provide. After months of constant trauma, we needed this token of good from our God! Oh, how we longed to see Him do this very uniquely for us, to reassure us of His presence and blessing in our lives. He had finally begun to break His silence, and the gifts began falling from above and around. Throughout the next few chapters, you will read lists of all of the financial gifts that we received. In perusing my journal, I noticed that the money stopped cold as soon as our need was ended. Our Jehovah-Jireh (the LORD will provide) is amazing!

March 3rd - *Handful of free medicine from nurse.*

March 5th - *$50 from a couple at church who said they hadn't been able to be at our house warming* **5 months ago!**

March 14th - *$50 from Grandmama for no special occasion.*

- $100 from someone at church

- Cashed in $50 savings bond (I'd had it since childhood, and we were desperate!)

24 – Let Him Bid Us Go, or Stay

I mentioned earlier that we were in limbo regarding whether or not we would be able to stay in Canada.

My journal speaks again with details of how God was working in our hearts concerning a move:

March 15 - *"This morning I studied Isaiah 22....The LORD gave me verses about being fastened and being still. He settled my heart and gave me peace about staying. The neat thing is that Jonathan has been reading verses in different places in the Bible, but has been impressed with the same theme. The LORD is settling both of our hearts that we should stay in Canada and trust Him."*

As impossible as it seemed that we would be able to stay, this is what we were led to tell the waiting deacons. We gave our answer to them shortly after the journal records this entry. On March 29, the church held a vote for whether or not to keep us on staff. It was 100% in favor for us to stay. God had provided in another area of our life, and we were thankful!

Meanwhile, financial gifts continued to trickle in during the month of March. And nestled between the thoughtful gifts was a big surprise:

March 19th - *$20 from someone at church*

March 21st was an epic day- *I found a $500 mistake in our checkbook,* **in our favour.** Somehow we had forgotten to add in a $500 deposit. Seriously. That has NEVER happened again! My journal records that *even with buying medication, we broke even and didn't lose any money. Praise the LORD!*

March 30th - *Exchanged notecards with a visiting missionary. We both gave each other $20.*

March 31st - *$60 from Mom.*

April dawned, and continued to bring financial blessings for the ongoing costs of my medications. Here are my journal entries that were of a financial nature from that month:

April 2nd - *$200 from someone anonymously.*

April 3rd - *Got tax check for $845.*

April 9th - *$50 from someone anonymously.*

April 15th - *$50 from friends.*

April 16th - $20 from someone at church.

April 27th - $100 from Shining Light Baptist Church (the church where my husband did his college internship). We have no idea how they knew of our need, and there was no explanation in the envelope— just the love gift.

April also records the monumental fact that, *"people are starting to say I look pregnant."* It was about time! I started the month at 24 weeks along, and was gradually gaining strength. I had even been able to go on a youth group trip to Halifax for a weekend. I was heavily medicated and exhausted easily, but I managed to be up and around. I was now able to eat more of a variety of foods, and always had some little bags of emergency snack foods or fruit in my purse. I would describe my physical state at this point in my pregnancy as being "normal morning sickness." While most women are happily enjoying their pregnancy at 24 weeks, with morning sickness long behind them, I felt like the pregnancy had just begun in terms of what normal morning sickness should be like. However, it was fabricated by medications, and my body was well aware of that. Just a few missed doses could land me in the hospital again. Each time I was tempted to skip my meds because I felt ok (I desperately wanted to slash the cost of the Zofran!), my husband gently encouraged me to stay on the full dose. It was working, after all, so why rock the boat?

Because my health was finally improving, my husband was able to dedicate more time to his church ministry duties. I kept a low profile at home, and only occasionally took a few outings to our beach (which was literally our backyard) and to town.

My journal entry from April 22, garnishes the memory of an outing that, for once, did not involve anything medical:

"Shopping in Yarmouth. For once we did something there besides go to the hospital! We got the baby's carseat and stroller. It still doesn't seem real that we're having a baby."

25 – Pregnant Women Shopping and a Calico Cat

The trauma of the past five months had begun to settle in heavily, and some aspects continued even after the baby's birth. Simple tasks were suddenly a great joy for me to perform. It was exhilarating to make it through a hot shower and be able to do my own hair. I looked forward to cooking a meal, doing laundry and housework, and being able to step outside and breathe in deeply the fresh ocean air.

I felt like I was on top of the world the first time I went shopping for groceries. I thoroughly enjoyed pushing my own cart and I soaked in the sight of the brightly colored produce and food packages. I felt completely out of touch with normal life- almost like I had stepped into a timeline where I didn't belong because I had been absent for so long.

During those days and for months after this, whenever I saw a pregnant woman shopping, I caught myself gawking at her. *"You mean,"* I gasped in my brain, *"She is pregnant and she is **shopping?!**"* I honestly could not fathom being happily pregnant and being able to go on a fun outing. I always needed to know where a chair was if I felt faint, where the washroom was if I needed to be sick, and where my stash of meds were if I needed a boost to make it through the outing.

It was dawning on me that I was definitely not experiencing a normal pregnancy. If only I had known that I never would experience that, it might have been easier to accept. Instead, I still clung to the hope that the days ahead would bring "fluffy" feelings, leaving me disappointed day by day to find that I was still too weak to lead a normal life.

I was still very weak and spent a lot of time resting. I started wishing for something to cuddle...and my husband agreed to let me get a cat.

We began watching the paper for free kittens, and one day we saw an attractive ad. We drove out to the home and chose a kitten—a calico that we still have today, almost seven years later. We named her BoPeep and she became my resting companion. Whenever I went to the couch, she followed and curled up in the corner of my tummy. She would wake up and purr when she felt the baby move. She is still an amazing animal with children. I wasn't sure how she would do when the baby was born, but she decided to "own" him. Only one time did I think about getting rid of her when I found her in his crib. But she never hurt him. In fact, she cried when he cried, and when we got a babysitter, she walked the hallway meowing. Her baby was gone. Two and a half years later when we brought baby sister home, Bo walked over to the carseat and sniffed our girlie. She turned her nose into the air and walked away. The boy was her baby! She is unbelievably patient as she lets the kids dress her in crazy outfits and carry her upside down. When they sit on her, she rolls out from under them and walks away. BoPeep is one of the best choices we've ever made!

26 – Milestones

May was a month of milestones for our little family. God continued to bring in financial gifts through the most unexpected ways.

May 1st - *Immigration Canada granted us both 3-year visas! They also returned the $150 we paid in fees. Praise the LORD for this progress towards permanency in the country!*

May 5th - *$100 more from Shining Light Baptist Church.*

May 10th - *$155 more from tax return (I have no idea why our tax money came in spurts that year, but it sure helped!)*

May 15th - *$25 in an anniversary card from our pastor and his wife back in North Carolina.*

May 14, was our first wedding anniversary. What a wild ride of a year it had been. Never did we imagine on our wedding day that the "in sickness and in health" part of our vows would be tested so soon, and so long.

On this, our first anniversary, we started a tradition of going away for a few days each year to celebrate together. We hadn't even had time to explore our area, having only explored the area hospitals—ha!

But we found what looked like a cozy little spot in Annapolis Royal, Nova Scotia. We rented a cabin on a lake and did a little bit of "roughing it." We still had electricity, but we cooked over a fire, and had a rather primitive washroom. The first day brought the most adventure that my pregnant self could handle—canoeing. I grew up canoeing often, but hadn't done it in a while. We braved the fog and rather chilly temps to take a skim around the lake. My poor husband had never canoed before, so he was making me nervous. Besides that, I kept having horrible daydreams that involved envisioning me falling to the bottom of the lake. I do *not* know how to swim, and the farther out we went the more my panic grew. My sweet husband soon took me back to the shore and he went back out by himself. For the next few days, we contented ourselves with games and long conversations by the fireplace, with one outing into "town" to visit the gardens.

On the final day of our trip, we walked an easy trail at Kejimkujik and enjoyed the waterfalls.

Our trip was slightly complicated by the fact that (a) I had to be near a washroom at all times and I had to stay on top of my medications, and (b) our newly adopted kitten, BoPeep, was not yet old enough to be home alone. So we brought her with us...and her litter pan...and her car carrier...and her food...and her water...and her treats...and her toys.

Yeah, it was a bit of an ordeal. And when we went into town, we had to make sure she wasn't in the car too long, etc. It's rather humorous now as I look back on it. It was probably breaking us in to having a little one to care for!

27 – The Miraculous

Do you have times in your life that you will never forget because God answered prayer and performed a seemingly impossible miracle in your life? We do, and one of them happened during our experience with HG. It ended up being one of the most tangible ways that we saw God's hand in our then crazy, non-sensical lives.

The month of June arrived and brought more monetary gifts that encouraged us as the bills continued to mount and the calls from doctors and hospitals continued to oppress. We figured that this was the way God has chosen to answer our prayers and help us pay off our bills. Little by little, we told ourselves. Someday we'll get this thing paid off, and hopefully we'll still be alive to see it! My journal entry for June 1, sheds some light on our renewed spirits:

"Applied for MSI cards and coverage. Now all we can do is wait and continue to pray. Our God is able to work for us a miracle! We still owe over $50,000. It's impossible to pay at our measely $20 per month! We'll see what happens..."

June 4th - *$20 from a man in the church.*

June 5th - *$100 more from Shining Light Baptist Church. $25 in a birthday card from Mom.*

June 8th - *$25 in a birthday card from Grandmama.*

On June 9, just 8 days after our application for medical coverage, the epic **miracle occurred:**

We had applied for our MSI (Medical Services Insurance) cards from the province of Nova Scotia. Being temporary residents, we weren't completely sure if we would even qualify. But we did, and on this particular day we received our medical cards in the mail. Thereafter, I began showing my medical card at each doctor and hospital appointment, and it was accepted without any questions. (Only once did we have a doctor's wife insist that my card was not valid because it started with a "0", typical for the type of visa we held at the time. But she was wrong, and after a few calls even that bill was covered.)

But what was even more amazing is that the Nova Scotia MSI program decided to **back pay everything** from the day we stepped into the country (8 months earlier). This was very unexpected, as persons with our type of visa were not promised coverage or back pay. All of a sudden, in a moment, our $50,000 debt was wiped clean. Months of agonizing prayer were answered and our thankfulness knew no bounds! From that day on (further putting us in awe of how God works), we didn't receive a single financial gift until early August, when MSI began to **refund** all of our paid increments of money to different doctors and hospitals. Then the envelopes began to trickle in with **checks** in them instead of bills. We ended up not having to pay for any of my care except for my medications and the ambulance rides that had not been doctor ordered. The cost of those still came out of pocket, and still cost several thousand dollars by the time I had the baby, but it paled in comparison to the cost of the hospitalizations!

Psalm 118:23 became a favourite verse to quote when we were overwhelmed at God's goodness to us: *"This is the LORD's doing; it is marvelous in our eyes."*

My journal entry for June 9, sums up what we were feeling (bear with all of the exclamation points I used on that day):

"This is a day never to be forgotten! We got our MSI cards in the mail, as well as some refund money and statements that our medical bills are covered! We simply have to call and apply my number to the bills. They back paid every cent of our owed $50,000 from the

'day we entered the country.' Our hearts are full and overflowing—God has truly worked a miracle for us! Praise God for answered prayer!"

One bill remained that we weren't sure about being covered. It was the ambulance bill from when I was transferred from Yarmouth to Halifax. That bill alone was $900. We decided to call about it, and after having it confirmed that the ambulance was indeed doctor ordered, that bill was also paid in full. What a week!

28 – Time to Wait

By late June, I was frequently having false labor. I had had Braxton Hicks contractions since I was 13 weeks along, so I knew what those felt like. But I began having episodes of stronger, regular contractions that sent us to the hospital several times, only to have us return home after a few hours of observation. Nothing was happening. It was still a bit early (I was around 35 weeks along) so I was sent home on "almost bed rest." A week of mostly resting and very limited activity left me stir crazy, after already having spent months in bed. I was ready for this awful ordeal to be over!

Our church Vacation Bible School was coming up shortly, and one of the ladies who was organizing it asked me if I would like to help her do some cutting for the crafts she was preparing. Of course I would—it would give me something to do! She brought over a pile of laminated circles with verses on them, and I began cutting. Maybe I'm a slow learner, because I was about half finished cutting one set of verses before I realized what verse I was cutting! My faithful journal records:

June 25th - *Home again on rest. I've been cutting out verses for VBS. What verse do you suppose I've been cutting? About 50 circles that say, 'Wait on the LORD.' Ok, I get the message. It's not yet time for Baby."*

July arrived and so did several of my due dates. When I say "several" it's because it seemed that every time I went to an appointment, the doctor changed my due date. I was seeing a rotation of six doctors in the prenatal clinic along with my specialist. They never could agree, so I wasn't really able to keep a fixed date in my mind. It's just as well, though, since all of the dates I had been given came and went with no baby. July kept us busy, though, and I was so ready for baby that I embraced busy and ditched the idea of rest. It was now safe for baby to come, so I worked with gusto. A team from Greenville, SC, came up to our church to run our VBS. There was much prep work to be done, as well as cooking for and hosting the team. We had a great week, and ended the VBS with a daily high of 81 children in attendance!

The team left on a Monday, and right before they left one of the older team members handed my husband a wad of money. It was $100. Once again we were humbled and thankful for God's continued provision for us. About a week after that, we were in the grocery store in line waiting to pay. A random woman in front of us turned and handed us $40 to help pay for our groceries! Random to us, but planned by our generous and loving God! Keep in mind that we were still paying for my medications (and would be paying those off for years to come) so even though the financial gifts had slowed down, we were ever grateful and still needful of each one God sent our way.

On July 24, I hit the 40-week mark. I hit rock bottom too, emotionally. My husband came home a few times to find me in a puddle of tears, convinced that I contained the only baby in the world that would never be born! If you've experienced those "end of pregnancy" hormones, you know what I mean.

July 27 sent me back to the hospital with regular contractions. I still had not dilated, though, and after several hours of assessment, the doctor told me I could stay the night, but that if I hadn't begun to dilate by morning, he was sending me home again. How. We. Prayed!

Morning dawned and guess what? I was at 3 cm. Not much, but enough to keep me there. We waited all day for things to progress more, but it was more of nothing. By Saturday, even the doctor agreed that it was time to do something. Although they still didn't consider me overdue (I did, though, by my dates!), they gave us the option of induction.

My husband and I were not thrilled at the thought of induction, especially considering that I would be forced to have an epidural along with the procedure.

We talked, prayed, and weighed our options. And we decided to go ahead with the induction. It would be the next day, so we had some time to enjoy each other and our last day of being a family of two.

The hospital granted us a day pass so we could go into town for a while. Possibly, the nurse said, things would get going on their own while I was out. Then I could just come back and have the baby – so easy, right? I wish!

So I put on normal clothes instead of hospital gowns and normal shoes instead of plastic slippers. We went out to eat, calling it our "last supper." It was such a weird feeling, after nine months of trauma and uncertainty, to KNOW that our baby was going to be born the next day. I couldn't wrap my head around it. We talked about whether it would be a girl or a boy (we still had the gut feeling that it was a girl), and made sure we were settled on the names we had chosen.

After we ate, we went to a department store and bought an exercise ball to use during labor. I didn't realize that I would be numb from the chest down, so I never got to use the ball. We ended up taking it home with us and it deflated on its own shortly after.

Later that evening after rambling around until we were tired, we headed back to the hospital for our last night before becoming parents. We called our parents to tell them the plan. Jonathan had a funny "tradition" for when he made calls using our phone cards (which we used all the time since our calls were international). He would say the first string of numbers and then add a sing-song rhyme to go along with it, like this: "3, 4, 2, 9; Our little baby's gonna be just fine! 2, 5, 6, 8; Our little baby had better appreciate!" It always made me laugh.

29 – Labor Day

I was monitored through the night, so we didn't get much sleep. I arose in the morning and took a bath, during which my nurse came in and declared that I "had better eat a big breakfast." I was a bit nervous, so I wasn't very hungry, but I managed to get something substantial down. I shouldn't have bothered—I saw it again during labor.

Around 11:00 AM, the anesthesiologist came in to administer my epidural. I was probably the most nervous about this part. My mom had an epidural with my sister, and ended up with a terrible spinal headache afterwards. I was leery of epidurals to begin with, but in my case, they didn't give me a choice. So over I bent and waited for something...I didn't know what to expect. The doctor who administered it didn't exactly help to ease my nerves. I was shaking hard and he was trying to get me to be still. He kept shouting, "Do you feel pain?! Do you feel pain?!" I didn't know if I was supposed to feel pain or not. I didn't feel any, so he proceeded.

I definitely wasn't prepared for my whole body to feel paralyzed. The nurses had to turn me and put me back on the bed. I panicked and it took me a few minutes to calm down as I realized that the "I can't move" feeling was normal. However, I froze all the way up to the base of my neck. It felt hard to breathe all of a sudden, and my blood pressure bottomed out. I almost fainted, but instead I got sick. I was unbearably hot, though shaking, so cold washcloths were kept on my neck, head, and chest.

Labor began to progress rather quickly, and consequently the nurse withdrew the medication from my IV so that I would be able to push when it was time. I also received a catheter, which I have heard can be painful. I didn't feel a thing since I was numb. But I developed a bladder infection after the birth, so I guess I paid my dues.

My husband laughs when we talk about my being in labor. I was expecting him to be a little squeamish, thinking that he would pass out or not be able to stay in the room. As I noticed lunchtime coming and then going, I said, "Honey, you must be hungry. Go get something to eat." But he assured me he was fine.

I should interject something about our wonderful doctor. He was Dr. B, one of six doctors in the prenatal clinic. He had been our favorite all along, and we hoped he would be on call when I went into labor. I began to pray that he would be. And God answered, for on the morning of my scheduled induction, he came on call. My labor progressed faster than he expected, and once when he came in to check me and realized where I was at, he said, "Well, guess I better get dressed." He was wearing a T-shirt and jeans, sipping his coffee. After he suited up, he began to tell stories in his casual, funny way. Upon hearing of my blood pressure incident, he said, "You know, you wouldn't make a very good astronaut. You see, when astronauts..." And he went on and on with a tale of astronauts. I didn't comprehend half of it, being in the middle of a contraction. He had a wonderful way of putting us at ease. He'd been sympathetic all through the pregnancy, and we'd come to know him more personally than any of the other doctors. I should add that my specialist was supposed to deliver me, but about a month before my due date, he scheduled a trip back to Africa. At the time, it was frustrating to be shifted into the clinic rotation at the last minute, but it turned out to be part of our answer to prayer for Dr. B to be our delivery doctor.

At 3:11 PM, after about an hour of pushing, our baby was born. He weighed 8 pounds, 7 ounces. I'll never forget my husband's response of shock. He gasped, "It's a boy!" I was shocked too. Our intuition had been wrong all along.

I held Caleb Joel right away, and I would be lying if I told you that all of the sweet feelings of motherhood washed over me. They didn't. After all of the trauma of the past almost year, I didn't know how to feel. I was just so glad to NOT be pregnant any longer. It was confusing to finally see what I had been trying to imagine all along, without success. And my body. Oh, it was so weak and so depleted. How was I going to take care of this baby who needed still more from me?

After the birth, Dr. B gave Jonathan his famous "placenta tour." It was fascinating for him, and although I only saw a quick glimpse of it, Jonathan told me about it later. Turns out, he wasn't squeamish at all!

We finally got settled into our room around 7:00 PM. I had to remain on my back for 24 hours to reduce the chance of developing the spinal headache. I thought I was home free after that, so I timidly rose from my bed and took a bath. After the bath, I settled into a rocking chair to hold my baby. I held him for fewer than ten minutes, for gradually as I sat, a pounding headache began. In record time, the pain was unbearable and I was back in bed, calling for relief. Dr. B could only let me have Tylenol, since I was attempting to nurse (mistake #1). I ended up with a nasty nurse who forced Caleb into me to nurse. I was unable to help, so someone had to hold him there. It took him a long time to learn how to latch on—very frustrating for everyone involved.

As the hours passed, it became evident that I had indeed developed the spinal headache from leaking too much spinal fluid during the epidural insertion. By that evening, my head was covered in ice; that was the only way I could tolerate the pain. To call this simply a "headache" seems a bit unjust. If you've ever had a spinal headache, you know what I mean. It is a pain so intense and heavy unlike even a migraine, and much worse. It takes the human body a long time to make spinal fluid to replace what is lost. My doctor considered doing a blood patch to try to speed up the process, but in the end decided not to mess with it any more. The result was my having to tough it out.

The day after Caleb's birth, I was moved to a private room and we embarked on a long week of pain and struggle. This was a difficult time for me, considering that no one had prepared me for how grueling recovery from childbirth could be. Even if I hadn't had the headache, there were other things that were shocking and very painful to me. Caleb and I did not bond. How could we? Jonathan did all of the changings and hall-walkings. He held him while the nurse pricked his foot. Caleb had a cry that sounded exactly like the meow of a cat. It was so cute, yet sad for me to hear.

I was in the hospital for ten days after Caleb's birth, flat on my back. It was extremely hard emotionally and by the tenth day I was begging my doctor to let me go home. He consented under one condition: that I would have round-the-clock help until the headache subsided. We agreed, and soon packed up to go home.

Once home, I found my place on the couch and hardly moved for many days. My mom flew in to Halifax soon after and Jonathan went to pick her up. She stayed 2 ½ weeks, during which I began to recover under her nutritious meals and constant help. Caleb was about three weeks old when the headache finally completely subsided. I began to notice that each day the pain was slightly less until it was gone. My back stayed painful for months afterward, but I was immensely relieved to be free of that awful head pain. I think I'd rather go through labor again than have a headache like that again.

Because my medications were antiemetics, I had to remain on them even after the birth and gradually wean off of them. I hated taking a pill that I felt I didn't need anymore (especially given the cost) but I knew I'd have to endure the withdrawal without them. And I was often still very nauseated without them. Although I was nursing, I continued on the main pill (Zofran) until I was only taking a quarter of a pill. Eventually I was med free and oh, what a blessing that was to our bank account!

I continued nursing Caleb until he was eight months old. However, we noticed that he was not gaining weight properly. As in, he didn't double his birth weight until he was one year old. One day when he was eight months old and some odd days, I pumped out some milk so we could go out. The milk looked like water. I was shocked. My body was so incredibly weak from the pregnancy that it couldn't even make milk. We had to figure out a different way. I disliked nursing anyway; it was always very painful and not a bonding time at all. To me it was just "feeding my baby" and I wished for an easier way. One day in particular I got bitten (Caleb got his first tooth at three months old) and then a few minutes later, he had a blow-out diaper. I was reading a paperback book while nursing. Guess what happened to the book? It was unsalvageable, so into the garbage it went. It was just one more reason to be done with nursing.

We went on a little trip to Moncton, New Brunswick, and visited friends of ours who had a baby boy Caleb's age (my friend and I were due the same week originally, but I went late). While there, I noticed her routine with formula and began to contemplate the possibility of bottle feeding. By the time we left, we were convinced that this was what our family needed, and even though finances were very tight, we had to find a way to make it work. God provided, and we switched Caleb to formula. Thankfully, he did wonderfully on the store brand, and our whole family was happier!

Conclusion – I Gave Birth to More Than A Baby

As a Hyperemesis survivor, I see birth a little differently than some. I fit into a small category (1-2%) of women who suffer with this life-threatening and life-changing disease. *When we give birth to our babies, we give birth to more than a baby.*

• What are some of the things we give birth to? Well, for starters, we give birth to a new normal. Life has changed forever in so many ways. Emotionally, we are devastated by disappointed dreams. Physically, we have a long road to walk to enjoy health again. We give birth to the possibility of healing. In a practical sense, we give birth to financial relief, to being able to live somewhat medication-free. Let me share a list of some of the most profound things in my life that I gave birth to the day I gave birth to my son:

- The ability to eat a full meal (a small one at that, since my stomach had shrunk significantly).
- The luxury of drinking a tall glass of cold water—oh, the bliss! I still to this day cannot drink water without thinking of the days when I would have given my very life to be able to chug a glass of water.
- The blessing of getting through a day without having to fear getting sick.
- The hope of a healthy child.
- The ability to do housework.
- The endurance to take a hot shower and dry my own hair.
- The comfort of being able to tolerate my husband next to me in bed (instead of him being on the floor!)
- Being able to sleep through the night (not having to wake up and keep the medication schedule going).
- The stamina to get ready for church or another outing, and still have the strength to attend and enjoy the outing.
- The fun of going shopping by myself (actually this took a while to incorporate back into my life).
- The ability to drive again (and ride without hating every bump).

- The pleasure of cooking a meal for my husband.
- Being able to sit up and read or watch a movie for more than ten minutes at a time.
- The endurance to be on my feet for more than a few seconds without collapsing.
- The comfort of lying in bed without the intense pain of bed sores.
- The luxury of enjoying "normal" life again.

There are many, many more "little" things that I know I took for granted before my pregnancy. Truthfully, I have done it since then. But having survived HG has been a lasting life lesson in enjoying the small gifts that God gives me each day.

Hyperemesis Gravidarum is a condition that affects women not just physically, but emotionally, mentally, and spiritually. Recovery is often slow and painful; therefore, continued support is crucial even after the pregnancy is over and life seemingly settles back into a normal routine. After HG, many things are never the same again. There is hope, and there is support out there!

When my son was a few months old, our local paper ran an article about a Canadian woman who was running for the cause of HG. I was shocked to find that others knew about this condition, and a ray of hope was born in my heart. Maybe there was someone who understood. I found out that there were many more than one someone- there was a whole support forum waiting with open arms to help HG moms survive. The newspaper article cited the website *www.helpher.org* as a forum for women with HG. I joined immediately and was part of that amazing support group for several years. They are dedicated and active in the lives of many women. I highly recommend HG sufferers and family members to read the valuable information on this site.

If you are suffering with HG, you don't have to suffer alone. If you are a family member or friend who is trying to support someone with HG, do some research. Be the best support that that precious woman has in her life right now. Her life and the life of her baby depend on it.

www.ingramcontent.com/pod-product-compliance
Lightning Source LLC
Chambersburg PA
CBHW070925290526
45795CB00001B/420